Copyright 2023

All right reserved.No part of this book should be reproduced without express permission of the author.

Reproduction of all or any part of this book is punishable unders relevant law.

Table of Contents

Being constipated means your bowel movements are tough or happen less often than normal. Almost everyone goes through it at some point.

Although it's not usually serious, you'll feel much better when your body is back on track.

The normal length of time between bowel movements varies widely from person to person. Some people have them three times a day. Others have them just a few times a week.

Going longer than 3 or more days without one, though, is usually too long. After 3 days, your stool gets harder and more difficult to pass.

BREAKFAST

1. Shirred Eggs with Leeks

Prep Time: 10 Minutes

Cook Time: 20 Minutes

Servings: 6

Ingredients

- 2 tablespoons salted butter, plus more for greasing
- 1 large red bell pepper, thinly sliced
- 1 leek, trimmed and minced
- 1 bunch green onions, white and light green parts only, minced
- 6 large eggs
- 12 tablespoons heavy cream
- ½ teaspoon sea salt
- ¼ teaspoon freshly cracked black pepper
- 2 ounces freshly grated Parmesan cheese
- Chopped fresh flat-leaf parsley and/or chives, for serving

- Crusty bread, for serving

Instructions

1. Preheat the oven to 375°F. Grease 6 ramekins with butter and arrange them on a rimmed baking sheet.

2. Melt the butter in a small skillet over medium heat. Add the bell pepper, leek, and green onion. Cook, stirring occasionally, until the bell pepper is tender, about 6-7 minutes.

3. Divide the mixture evenly among the prepared ramekins, creating a small well in each one. Carefully crack one egg into each well, then top each egg with 2 tablespoons of the heavy cream. Season with salt and pepper, then sprinkle on some of the Parmesan.

4. Bake until the egg whites are barely set and yolks are still runny, 10 to 15 minutes. (The eggs will continue to cook after they come out of the oven). Garnish with parsley and/or chives, if desired. Serve warm with crusty bread alongside.

Prep Time: 25 Minutes

Cook Time: 10 Minutes

Servings: 3

Ingredients

- 4 thick bacon slices, cut into 1-inch pieces, optional
- 1 Tbsp Extra virgin olive oil
- 1/2 small yellow onion, diced, about 1/2 cup
- 2 garlic cloves, minced
- 4 cups roughly chopped Swiss chard leaves, stems removed, about 1 bunch
- 1/2 cup pitted castelvetrano olives, pitted, sliced, plus more for garnish
- 2/3 cup heavy cream
- 4 eggs
- 1 Tbsp salted butter or olive oil
- 1/4 cup panko
- 1/4 cup crumbled feta
- 1/2 tsp flaky salt for finishing
- 2 Tbsp minced chives for garnishing
- 1 loaf of crusty bread, for serving

Instructions

1. Heat the oven to 425°F.

2. In a medium sized ovenproof skillet, cook the bacon over medium heat. Transfer the bacon to a paper towel lined plate. Drain off all but 1 tablespoon of the bacon grease.

3. Add 1 tablespoon of olive oil to the pan. Still over medium heat, add the onions, cooking until beginning to soften, about 5 minutes. Add the garlic and swiss chard, continuing to cook until the chard begins to wilt about 2-3 more minutes. Return the cooked bacon to the pan along with the olives. Remove from heat.

4. Create 4 wells in the chard mixture. This is where you will crack the eggs. Once all of the eggs are in the wells you created, drizzle the entire dish with the cream. Place the dish in the oven and cook for 8-10 minutes. Just until the white parts of the eggs are no longer transparent, but the egg yolks are still runny.

5. While the eggs are baking, melt the butter in a small skillet, over medium heat. Add the panko and toss to combine with the butter. Continue cooking and tossing until the panko is golden brown before removing from the heat.

6. Remove the eggs from the oven and sprinkle the toasted panko over the entire dish. Sprinkle with the feta, extra olives (if desired), flaky salt and fresh chives.

7. Serve alongside some good toasted bread.

Prep Time: 15 Minutes

Cook Time: 25 Minutes

Servings: 4

Ingredients

- Seasoned Cabbage:
- 2 cups finely shredded green cabbage
- 1 tablespoon vegetable or extra virgin olive oil
- 1 tablespoon white vinegar
- ½ teaspoon sea salt
- ⅛ teaspoon black pepper
- ½ teaspoon taco seasoning

Tortilla chips:

- 1/4 cup vegetable oil, for frying
- 8 corn tortillas, cut into 8 wedges each
- 1/2 teaspoon sea salt
- 1 cup salsa verde, homemade or store bought

Crema:

- ¼ cup sour cream

- 1 tablespoon heavy cream or milk
- 2 teaspoon lime juice
- 1 teaspoon taco seasoning

For Serving:

- 4 fried eggs
- avocado or guacamole
- queso fresco, crumbled
- hot sauce
- jalapeños, thinly sliced or pickled
- raw onion, white or red onion, thinly sliced
- cilantro, minced

Instructions

1. Make the seasoned cabbage. In a medium bowl mix together cabbage, olive oil, vinegar, salt, pepper and taco seasoning, toss until combined. Set aside.

2. To make the tortilla chips start by placing a large skillet over medium-high heat, add the oil. When the oil is glistening, add 1/2 of the tortilla wedges and cook until lightly browned on each side, about 1-2 minutes. Using tongs, transfer the tortilla chips to a paper towel lined plate. Sprinkle lightly with 1/4

teaspoon salt. Repeat this process with remaining tortillas, adding a little more oil if needed.

3. Drain the oil from the pan. Add the salsa to the pan and heat until warmed through, about 2 minutes. Add all the chips back into the pan. Stir carefully to coat the chips in the salsa without breaking them. Cook until the tortillas are heated through, and slightly softened, about 3 minutes. Taste and season with salt as needed.

4. In a small bowl mix together the sour cream, heavy cream or milk, lime juice and taco seasoning until fully combined.

5. Serve the chilaquiles warm, topped with crema, fried eggs, seasoned cabbage and your favorite garnishes: avocado or guacamole, queso fresco, hot sauce, jalapeños, white or red onion or cilantro.

6. To make this a more hearty meal, serve with pulled chicken or warmed pinto beans.

Prep Time: 15 Minutes

Cook Time: 20 Minutes

Servings: 6

Ingredients

- 1/3 cup cream cheese, room temperature
- 1 tsp tomato paste, from a tube (that way you don't waste a whole can)
- 1 1/4 tsp fine sea salt
- 2 pinches garlic powder
- 2 pinches onion powder
- 6 multigrain tortillas or wraps (10 inch)
- cooking spray
- 12 eggs (whites only)
- 1 (5 oz) box baby spinach, about 4 cups
- 2 oz sun-dried tomatoes, about 10 from an oil packed jar, finely chopped
- 2 oz feta, crumbled
- pepper to taste

Instructions

1. In a small bowl mix together the cream cheese, tomato paste, 1/4 teaspoon salt, 1 pinch garlic powder and 1 pinch onion powder until smooth.

2. Spread the tomato cream cheese onto the center of the tortillas, dividing evenly.

3. In a medium bowl whisk the egg whites together with remaining 1 teaspoon salt, 1 pinch garlic powder and 1 pinch onion power until smooth.

4. Spray a medium non-stick skillet, with cooking spray and set it over medium heat. When the skillet is hot, add the spinach and cook until wilted, about 5 minutes. Divide the spinach evenly between the tortillas, placing it on top of the cream cheese, along with the feta and sun-dried tomatoes.

5. Spray the skillet again with cooking spray and cook the egg whites, gently pushing them around the pan until mostly firm, about 5 minutes. Divide the eggs between the tortillas.

6. Wipe out the skillet and spray with cooking spray. Alternatively you can heat a panini press to medium heat. Fold each wrap up like a burrito so that the ends are tucked and none of the filling will fall out. Place them into the skillet or panini press as many will fit at

a time. Cook until golden brown on both sides, about 4-6 minutes total.

Prep Time: 1hrs 15 Minutes

Cook Time: 45 Minutes

Servings: 8

Ingredients

Filling:

- 1 small sweet onion, halved and thinly sliced
- 1 tbsp butter
- 1 tsp brown sugar
- 6 large eggs
- 3/4 cup heavy cream
- 1 tsp salt
- 1/2 tsp fresh ground black pepper
- 2-3 oz Parmigiano-Reggiano cheese finely grated
- 1 medium heirloom tomato, chopped
- 2 garlic cloves, minced
- 1 handful of basil leaves, thinly sliced

Crust:

- 1 1/2 cup all purpose flour
- 9 tbsp unsalted butter, cold, 1/2 inch diced

- 1/2 tsp salt
- 3 1/2 tbsp ice water

Instructions

1. Before preparing quiche filling, dice 9 tablespoons of butter, place on parchment paper and put in freezer.
2. Melt the remaining butter in a small frying pan over medium-low heat until foaming. Add the onions and sugar, let them cook, stirring occasionally, until they are deep golden brown and caramelized, about 40 minutes. Add garlic to the pan and let them cook 5 minutes longer. Season well with salt and pepper, remove from the pan, and let cool.
3. While onions are caramelizing, place flour and ½ teaspoon salt into a food processor with fitted blade. Pulse to combine. Add the butter from the freezer. Pulse 8 to 12 times, until the butter is the size of peas. With the machine running, pour the ice water down the feed tube and pulse the machine until the dough begins to form a ball. Dump out on a floured board and roll into a ball.
4. Preheat oven to 375° F.

5. While onions are cooling, press dough into an 8 or 9 inch pie or quiche pan. Place in refrigerator while preparing the eggs.

6. Combine eggs, cream, salt and pepper in a food processor or blender. Blend the ingredients for 1 minute. Layer the tomatoes, cheese and basil in the bottom of the crust lined quiche pan. Evenly disperse onion and garlic over top, then pour the egg mixture on top of that. Bake for 35-45 minutes until the egg mixture is set. Cut into 8 wedges.

Prep Time: 15 Minutes

Cook Time: 18 Minutes

Servings: 6

Ingredients

- 2 tbsp olive oil
- 4 cups spinach leaves
- 8-10 asparagus spears, ends trimmed, thick ones cut in 1/2 lengthwise.
- 8 eggs
- 1/2 tsp sea salt
- 1/4 tsp freshly ground pepper
- 2 cups gruyere or comte, grated
- 3 tbsp fresh dill, finely chopped
- 2 tbsp fresh chives, finely chopped
- 8 oz Crème Fraîche

Instructions

1. Preheat oven to 375°F.

2. In a 10" nonstick, ovenproof skillet (such as cast iron) heat olive oil over medium heat. Add spinach and asparagus and cook until spinach has wilted. The asparagus will not be fully cooked. Turn off heat and remove asparagus and set aside on a plate.

3. In a medium bowl whisk eggs with salt and pepper. Carefully pour the eggs into the hot pan over the spinach. Layer the asparagus on the eggs, followed by the cheese, dill and then finally chives.

4. Bake the frittata for 12-18 minutes, or until eggs are cooked through.

5. Slice like a pie and serve with extra chives and a dollop of creme fraiche.

Prep Time: 20 Minutes

Cook Time: 55 Minutes

Servings: 8

Ingredients

- 1 Tbsp salted butter
- 1/2 medium onion, chopped
- 1 tsp Brown sugar
- 2 Garlic cloves, minced
- 6 Large eggs, room temperature
- 3/4 cup Heavy cream, room temperature
- 1 cup shredded cheese (Gruyère or sharp cheddar)
- 1 cup cooked, crumbled bacon or diced ham
- 1 tsp Sea salt
- 1/2 tsp Fresh ground black pepper
- 1/4 tsp ground nutmeg
- 1/2 recipe all-butter pie crust or one store bought pie crust

Instructions

1. Prepare your pie crust by rolling it out to 1/4-inch thickness and forming it in a pie plate or tart pan, chill in the fridge until ready to fill.

2. Preheat your oven to 375° F.

3. Melt the butter in a small skillet over medium heat. When the butter begins to foam, add the onions and brown sugar. Let them cook, stirring occasionally, until they are very tender, about 8-10 minutes. This is a good time to cook your bacon (in a separate skillet) if you are using bacon instead of ham. Add the garlic to the pan with the onions and cook 1 minute longer, until fragrant. Remove the skillet from the heat.

4. In a large bowl, whisk the eggs, cream, salt, pepper and nutmeg together until they're well combined. Stir in the cheese, bacon or ham, and the onion mixture. Pour the egg mixture into the prepared pie crust.

5. Bake for 35-45 minutes until the egg mixture is set and no longer jiggly in the center. Cut into 8 wedges.

Prep Time: 25 Minutes

Cook Time: 1hrs 15 Minutes

Servings: 8

Ingredients

- 1 loaf day-old baguette or crusty bread, crust removed, cut into 1 inch cubes
- 2 tbs butter
- 1 small onion
- 2 tbsp fresh thyme or rosemary (about 1 tbs)
- 8 oz mushrooms, sliced
- 3 cups fresh spinach, packed
- 2 cups swiss cheese, grated
- 8 eggs
- 2 cups whole milk
- 1 cup heavy cream
- 2 tsp kosher salt
- 1/2 tsp black pepper, freshly ground
- 1 tsp dijon mustard
- 1/4 tsp nutmeg, freshly grated

Instructions

1. Preheat oven to 400° F. Place the bread cubes on a baking sheet and toast in the oven until golden brown, about 10 minutes. Remove from the oven and set aside.

2. In a large sauté pan over medium heat, cook the onions, mushrooms and herbs in the butter until vegetables are softened, about 7 minutes. Add the spinach to the pan and cook another 5 minutes until the spinach is wilted and completely cooked down. Pull the pan off the heat, and let cool.

3. In a 9 inch square or round casserole (or a 9 inch springform pan) measure out the toasted bread. The amount of bread you need should fill the dish. Once you have measured this, place that amount of bread back into the empty mixing bowl. Add the onion mushroom mixture and 2 cups of swiss cheese to the bread in the mixing bowl. Toss to combine.

4. Turn oven down to 350° F.

5. In a blender combine the eggs, milk, cream, salt, pepper, mustard and nutmeg. Blend for 10 seconds until combined.

6. Line your dish with parchment paper or lightly grease the dish. Add the bread and mushroom onion mixture

to the pan. Carefully pour the egg mixture over the bread. Press the bread cubes down to make sure they are totally submerged. Note: This step can be made the night before.

7. Bake the strata uncovered until it has has puffed slightly, is golden brown on top and does not shimmy with uncooked egg mixture when you shake the pan, about 1 hour and 15 minutes. If the strata gets too dark, cover with foil and continue cooking. Let the strata cool in the pan on a wire rack for 15 minutes. Serve strata warm or at room temp.

Prep Time: 2hrs 30 Minutes

Cook Time: 15 Minutes

Servings: 12

Ingredients

- 2 cups whole milk
- 1/2 cup vegetable oil
- 1/2 cup sugar
- 2 tbsp almond extract
- 1 package active dry yeast
- 4 1/2 cups Bob's Red Mill Unbleached All-Purpose White Organic Flour
- 1/2 heaping tsp baking powder
- 1/2 scant tsp baking soda
- 1 1/2 tsp salt

Filling:

- 1 cup Tillamook Sweet Cream Butter (unsalted), softened
- 2 cups sugar
- 2 tsp Cardamom, ground

- Almond Glaze:
- 1 cup powdered sugar
- 1 tbsp whole milk
- 2 tsp almond extract

Instructions

1. Heat the milk, vegetable oil, sugar and almond extract in a medium saucepan over medium heat. (Do not allow the mixture to boil.) Set aside and cool. When mixture has cooled to 100-110°F, sprinkle the yeast on top and let it sit on the milk for 2 minutes.
2. Add 4 cups of the flour. Stir until just combined, cover the bowl with a clean kitchen towel, and set aside in a relatively warm place for an hour.
3. Remove the towel and add the baking powder, baking soda, salt and remaining ½ cup of flour. Stir thoroughly to combine. *Use the dough right away, or place in a mixing bowl and refrigerate for up to 3 days, punching down the dough if it rises to the top of the bowl.
4. Remove the dough from the bowl onto a floured surface, roll the dough into a large rectangle, about 30 x 10 inches.

5. In a small bowl, combine all filling ingredients until a soft paste is formed.

6. Using the back a spoon, evenly spread the filling to cover the entire surface of the dough.

7. Beginning at the end farthest from you, roll the rectangle tightly toward you. Use both hands and work slowly, being careful to keep the roll tight. When you reach the end, pinch the seam together. On a cutting board, using a sharp knife, make 1 ½-inch slices. 15-20 rolls.

8. Line a few baking dishes with parchment paper (alternatively, grease well with butter). Place the sliced rolls in the pans, being careful not to over crowd.

9. Preheat oven to 375° F. Cover rolls with a kitchen towel and set aside to rise on the countertop for at least 20 minutes before baking. Remove the towel and bake for 13 to 17 minutes, until golden brown. Don't let the rolls get overly brown.

10. In a bowl, whisk together the powdered sugar, milk and almond extract until very smooth. The icing should be thick but still pourable. If it is too thin add more sugar 1 tablespoon at a time. If it is too thick, add more milk ¼ teaspoon at a time.

11. After the rolls are finished baking, and still warm, generously drizzle icing over the top. Be sure to get it all around the edges and over the top. As they sit, the rolls will absorb some of the icing's moisture and flavor. It goes without saying that these are best served warm, but they are equally delicious even if made a day ahead.

Prep Time: 10 Minutes

Cook Time: 20 Minutes

Servings: 8

Ingredients

- 4 cups rolled oats
- 2 cups pecans, halves
- 1/4 cup chia seeds
- 1 cup pumpkin seeds
- 1 cup slivered almonds
- 1/4 cup sesame seeds
- 1 cup coconut flakes, sweetened or unsweetened
- 1/2 tsp salt
- 1 tsp cinnamon
- 1/2 cup coconut oil
- 1 tsp vanilla extract
- 1/4 cup real maple syrup, room temp
- 1 large egg white

Instructions

1. Preheat oven to 350°F. Line a small, rimmed baking sheet with parchment paper. Set aside.

2. Place rolled oats, pecans, chia seeds, pumpkin seeds, almonds, sesame seeds, coconut, salt and cinnamon in a large mixing bowl. Toss to combine.

3. In a separate small, microwave safe bowl, heat the coconut oil until liquified. You may also do this over the stove top using a small sauce or frying pan. Add the maple syrup and vanilla extract to the coconut oil. Pour coconut oil mixture into the oat mixture. Stir until coated evenly.

4. In separate small bowl beat the egg white until peaks have formed. Gently fold stiff egg white into the granola.

5. Carefully pour granola onto the rimmed baking sheet. Using the flat bottom of a glass cup, gently press granola into a solid, even layer. Bake for 20 minutes. Every oven is different and we recommend gently lifting the edge of the parchment paper ½ and ¾ of the way through to ensure none of the edges are getting too dark.

6. Let granola mixture cool for 10 minutes before breaking it apart. Store granola in an airtight container for up to 1 month.

11. Oat Scones

Prep Time: 15 Minutes

Cook Time: 15 Minutes

Servings: 8

Ingredients

- 1 1/2 cups flour
- 1 tsp baking powder
- 1/2 tsp baking soda
- 1/2 tsp salt salt
- 1/2 cup sugar
- 1/2 cup butter
- heaping 1/3 cup vanilla (or any flavor) yogurt
- 1 cup quick oats

Instructions

1. Preheat your oven to 375° F. In a mixing bowl combine the flour, baking soda, baking powder, salt and sugar. Stir dry ingredients until well combined.

Using a fork, pastry cutter or small knife, cut the butter into the dry ingredients. Once the butter is cut in and is the size of small pebbles add the yogurt. Combine until evenly dispersed and then add the quick oats. Mix with your hands until well incorporated.

2. On a parchment paper, use your hands to shape the dough into a circle that is ½ " thick. Cut the dough into 8 equal triangles and spread out onto the parchment paper.

3. Using a pastry brush, use a little bit of the yogurt to brush the tops of the prepared dough.

4. Bake on center rack of preheated oven for 15 minutes or until edges are golden brown. Allow to cool completely before serving. Enjoy!

Prep Time: 20 Minutes

Cook Time: 15 Minutes

Servings: 4

Ingredients

- 1.5 lb skirt or flank steak
- Salt
- Pepper
- 4 6" french or hoagie rolls, sliced in half diagonally
- 6 tbsp butter, softened
- 2 tsp garlic powder, granulated
- 2 cups grated gruyere or Swiss cheese
- minced parsley for garnish, optional
- 4 cups beef stock
- 1/4 tsp dried thyme
- 1 tsp salt
- 1 tsp sherry wine
- 1 tbsp Worcestershire
- 2 tsp garlic powder
- 2 tsp onion powder

Instructions

1. Heat a large cast iron skillet over high heat. Generously salt and pepper the steak and sear it until it reaches medium rare (135°F on an instant read thermometer), depending on thickness about 3 minutes each side. Let the steak rest for 5 minutes. Slice the steak into strips, as thin as possible against the grain and set aside.

2. In a medium sized saucepan set over medium heat, whisk the beef stock, dried thyme, salt, sherry, Worcestershire, garlic and onion powder, until fully combined. Simmer for 5 minutes.

3. Butter the inside of the each of the french or hoagie rolls and sprinkle with garlic powder and place them open faced on a rimmed baking sheet.

4. Turn oven broiler on medium. Quickly dip the strips of steak into the broth and place them in even amounts onto one side of each roll. Sprinkle ⅓ cup cheese on each sandwich and arrange them open face on the baking sheet.

5. Place the baking sheet under the broiler until cheese begins to melt, watching carefully for about 2 minutes. Remove from oven and sprinkle with parsley if desired.

6. In small cocottes or ramekins ladle ¾ cup serving of au jus into each container. Serve au jus with the warm sandwich.

Prep Time: 25 Minutes

Cook Time: 40 Minutes

Servings: 6

Ingredients

Salad:

- 4-6 eggs
- 4-6 oz pancetta, diced
- 1/2-1lb asparagus, woody ends trimmed
- salt and pepper to taste
- 6 oz spring lettuce mix
- 1 avocado
- 4 oz crumbled goat cheese
- 4 watermelon radishes, thinly sliced
- 1 cup sugar snap peas
- 1/4 cup sunflower seeds, roasted, salted
- 2 tbsp chives, minced

Dressing:

- 1 cup Extra virgin olive oil
- 1/3 cup white balsamic

- 1/4 cup lemon juice
- 1 garlic clove
- 1 tsp dijon mustard
- 1/2 cup loose packed basil
- 1/2 cup loosely packed mint
- 1 tbsp honey
- 1/2 tsp salt
- 1/4 tsp freshly ground black pepper

Instructions

1. Blend all ingredients for the dressing in a blender until smooth. Store in an airtight container until ready to use. Keep in refrigerator up to 2 weeks.

2. Cover the eggs with cool water by 1 inch. Slowly bring water to a boil over medium-high heat. When the water has reached a boil, cover with a tight fitting lid and remove the pan from the heat. Let sit 12 minutes. Transfer the eggs to a bowl of ice water to stop the cooking.

3. In a medium sized pan, sauté the pancetta until crispy. Drain onto a paper towel lined plate, reserving 2 teaspoons of fat in the pan. Place the asparagus into the still hot pan of pancetta fat. Sprinkle with a pinch

of salt and pepper. Sauté until tender, roughly 5-10 minutes. Set aside. Crack and peel the hard boiled eggs, slice them and set aside.

4. Spread the lettuce on a large platter. Top it in sections with the pancetta, asparagus, avocado, goat cheese, radishes, and peas. Sprinkle with chives and sunflower seeds. Serve alongside the herby dressing.

Prep Time: 35 Minutes

Cook Time: 25 Minutes

Servings: 8

Ingredients

- 1 lb Italian sausage
- 1 cup onion, diced
- 4 cloves garlic, roughly chopped
- 24 oz marinara sauce
- 14 oz tomato sauce
- 1 tsp salt
- 1 tbsp Italian seasoning
- ½ cup heavy cream
- 1 lb ziti pasta, cooked
- 8 oz fresh mozzarella, sliced
- 2 cups mozzarella cheese, shredded
- ¼ cup Parmesan cheese, grated
- ¼ tsp chili flakes
- 2 tbsp fresh basil, minced

Instructions

1. Preheat oven to 375°F

2. Cook the pasta al dente** in salted water. 1 pound of pasta = 1 tablespoon salt : 4 quarts (16 cups) water.

3. In a large dutch oven or soup pot set over medium-high heat. Brown the ground sausage, onion and garlic. Drain the fat if there is an excess of it.

4. Add the marinara sauce, tomato sauce, salt, Italian seasoning and heavy cream, stir until combined.

5. Drain the pasta, rinse it if it gets stuck together. Dump the pasta and 1 ½ cups shredded mozzarella cheese into the pot with the sauce. Stir to combine. Transfer the pasta and meat sauce to a 9X13 baking dish.

6. Add the fresh mozzarella slices to the top of the pasta along with the remaining ½ cup shredded mozzarella, cover and bake for 20 minutes. Remove the lid or foil and bake 5 more minutes until lightly browned and bubbling.

7. Remove from oven and sprinkle with parmesan, chili flakes and fresh basil.

8. The pasta should still have a bite to it, because it will continue cooking in the oven.

Prep Time: 20 Minutes

Cook Time: 15 Minutes

Servings: 6

Ingredients

- 1 lb cooked pasta of your choice, pasta water reserved
- 4 cups broccoli florets
- 2 cups basil leaves, lightly packed
- 2 garlic cloves
- ¼ cup pine nuts
- 1 cup extra virgin olive oil
- ½ tsp salt
- 1 cup Parmigiano-Reggiano, grated

Instructions

1. In a large pot bring water to a rapid boil.
2. Add the broccoli, bring the water back up to a boil for two minutes. Do not drain the water! Immediately transfer broccoli (with a slotted spoon) to a colander

place under cold running water to stop further cooking.

3. Bring the water back to a boil and add your favorite pasta and cook according to the package (reserve 1 cup of pasta cooking water before draining).

4. In a large blender or food processor, blend together broccoli, basil, garlic, pine nuts, olive oil, salt and Parmigiano-Reggiano until smooth. Slowly pour in 1 cup of reserved pasta water until a nice sauce is formed. If sauce is too thick, add more pasta water one tablespoon at a time.

5. Toss hot pasta with sauce until completely coated. Top with extra Parmesan, pine nuts and chili flakes if desired. Enjoy!

6. It is important to salt your water before adding the broccoli and pasta. Do this to your own taste.

Prep Time: 10 Minutes

Cook Time: 25 Minutes

Servings: 6

Ingredients

- 5 oz pancetta, diced
- 3 garlic cloves, minced
- 1 lb penne pasta
- 2 tbsp butter
- 2 tbsp flour
- 2 cups whole milk
- 4 oz goat cheese, crumbled, divided
- 1 tsp salt
- 1 ½ cups frozen peas, defrosted
- ¼ cup fresh chives, chopped

Instructions

1. Fry the pancetta in a large skillet set over medium heat. The time it takes for the pancetta to brown will depend on its size. Once the pancetta is turning

slightly brown, add the garlic. Sauté 1-2 minutes longer until the pancetta is crispy. Drain on a paper towel lined plate.

2. Add 4 quarts of water to a large pot set over high heat and bring to a boil. Once the water is boiling, salt it with two tablespoons of salt. Once the water returns to a boil add the pasta to the pot. Set a timer for 8 minutes (or the length of time called for on the pasta box).

3. While the pasta boils, make a garlicky béchamel sauce. In the skillet used for the pancetta, begin by melting butter over medium heat until it begins to bubble. Add the flour, and whisk to form a paste. Allow this butter-flour paste (also knowns as a roux) to cook, whisking constantly, for about 1 minute until the flour smell is gone. Add the milk in a slow, steady drizzle, whisking as you go.

4. Once all the milk has been added, turn the heat down to medium and stir constantly until sauce comes to a delicate simmer and thickens slightly. Reduce heat to low and cook, stirring, until sauce is thick enough to coat the back of a wooden spoon, about 3 minutes. Add 2 oz. crumbled goat cheese to the sauce and stir

until incorporated. Season with salt (and pepper if desired).

5. Drain your penne. Toss the cooked pasta into the finished béchamel along with the peas and the cooked pancetta/garlic. Salt to taste. Top the finished pasta with chives & the rest of the goat cheese. Enjoy.

Prep Time: 20 Minutes

Cook Time: 15 Minutes

Servings: 6

Ingredients

- 8 oz halloumi, 1/2 inch sliced
- 1 large avocado, 1/2 inch sliced
- olive oil
- 3 tbsp butter
- 1 cup panko bread crumbs
- 5 oz Arugula
- 1 pint cherry tomatoes, halved
- 1/2 cup Pickled onions

Creamy Basil Dressing:

- 1/3 cup Mayonnaise
- 1/4 cup Sour cream
- 1/2 tsp Dried parsley (or 2 tsp fresh)
- 1/2 tsp Onion powder
- 1/2 tsp Garlic powder
- 1/2 tsp Dried dill

- 1/4 tsp Salt
- 1/4 cup fresh basil, packed (2/3 oz)
- 1 tbsp milk, if needed

Instructions

1. Preheat a grill pan or outdoor grill to medium heat.
2. Brush the halloumi and avocado slices with olive oil. Place the avocado and halloumi on the grill until char marks appear, about 2 to 3 minutes each side.
3. Meanwhile make the dressing by combining all the ingredients in a small food processor and blending until smooth. Add milk only if needed for consistency.
4. In a medium skillet, melt the butter over medium heat. Add the panko to the butter and cook, tossing often until browned, about 4-5 minutes.
5. Place the arugula on a large platter. Add the tomatoes and onions. Sprinkle with the panko. Layer on the avocado and halloumi then drizzle with dressing.

Prep Time: 30 Minutes

Cook Time: 20 Minutes

Servings: 6

Ingredients

- 1/2 lb (8 oz) ciabatta or French bread, torn into 1-inch pieces
- 3 Tbsp Extra virgin olive oil
- 1/2 tsp salt
- 1/2 tsp granulated garlic powder
- 1 large shallot or 1/2 large red onion, thinly sliced
- 2/3 oz basil (1/4 cup chopped)
- 1 pint (10 oz) cherry tomatoes, cut in half and seeded
- 2 oz shaved parmesan cheese

Dressing

- 1/4 cup extra virgin olive oil
- 1 tsp honey
- 2 Tbsp white balsamic vinegar
- 1 large garlic clove, minced
- 1 tsp Dijon

- 1/4 tsp salt
- 1/4 tsp freshly ground black pepper

Instructions

1. Heat four cups of water to a boil and preheat the oven at 425°F.
2. In a medium bowl, whisk together all ingredients for the dressing until fully combined.
3. Place the shallots/onions into a fine mesh sieve set over the sink. Slowly pour the boiling water over them, quickly softening them as you go.
4. Add the softened onions to the bowl with the dressing, toss to combine
5. Place the bread on a large rimmed baking sheet and drizzle with 3 tablespoons olive oil, toss to evenly coat. Sprinkle with with 1/2 teaspoons salt and 1/2 teaspoons garlic powder toss to combine.
6. Bake in the oven for 10-12 minutes until golden brown all over.
7. In a large serving bowl, toss the toasted bread with the basil, tomatoes and parmesan. Drizzle the dressing over the bread/tomato mixture, tossing as you go, until fully combined.

Prep Time: 10 Minutes

Cook Time: 20 Minutes

Servings: 6

Ingredients

- 6 ears corn of corn, about 4 cups
- 1/4 cup finely diced radishes
- 1/2 bunch green onions, roughly chopped
- 1 Tbsp lime juice, from 1 lime
- 1/2 tsp sea salt
- 1/4 tsp freshly cracked black pepper
- 1/3 cup chipotle mayo
- 1/4 cup roughly chopped cilantro leaves
- 1/4 cup crumbled cotija cheese
- 1/4 tsp chipotle chili powder (or regular chili powder)

Instructions

1. To make this salad with Grilled Corn: Heat a grill on high for 10 min. Husk the corn, completely removing the silky hairs and lay the corn directly on the hot

grill. Once the corn begins to char, flip it to the other side. Continue flipping until the corn is charred on all sides, about 10 minutes total. Remove the corn from the grill and allow it to cool. Once the corn has cooled completely, use a sharp knife to remove the kernels from the corn.

2. To make this salad with Boiled Corn: Bring a large pot of water to a boil over high heat. Husk the corn, completely removing silky hairs. Boil the corn cobs for 8 minutes before removing them from the water, set aside to cool. Once the corn has cooled completely, use a sharp knife to remove the kernels from the corn.

3. To make this salad with Frozen Corn: In a large skillet, set over high, heat 1 tablespoon of vegetable oil over high heat. Add 4 cups of frozen corn and spread them out into a single layer. Allow the corn to cook over high heat until it begins to char. Stir corn and cook for another 2 minutes. Remove the pan from the heat and allow the corn to cool completely before using in the salad.

4. Assemble the salad:

5. In a medium sized bowl combine the corn kernels with the radishes, green onions, lime juice, salt and pepper. Toss the corn mixture with chipotle crema

until completely coated. Add a little more if desired. Sprinkle the salad with cilantro, cotija and chipotle powder.

Prep Time: 30 Minutes

Cook Time: 50 Minutes

Servings: 6

Ingredients

- 8 medium sized beets
- 4 tbsp olive oil
- 6 whole carrots, peeled, sliced into 2-inch pieces
- sea salt
- freshly ground pepper
- 2 cups watercress or spring salad mix
- micro greens, optional
- Green Goddess Dressing
- 4 oz goat cheese
- 1/3 cup olive oil
- 4 green onions, white and green parts
- 10 basil leaves
- 1/4 cup flat leaf parsley
- 1 garlic clove
- 1 tbsp fish sauce
- 1/4 cup freshly squeezed lemon juice

- 1/4 tsp freshly ground pepper
- 1/4 tsp sea salt

Instructions

1. Preheat oven to 375°F.
2. Trim the green tops off the beets. Place each beet on a square of tin-foil. Drizzle with a little olive oil and wrap the foil around the beet loosely, but making sure it is completely sealed. Place all the foiled wrapped beets on a baking sheet and roast for 45-50 minutes.
3. While the beets are roasting, place the carrots on a baking sheet and lightly drizzle with olive oil. Season the carrots with salt and pepper and roast in the over with the beets for the last 15-20 minutes.
4. Once the beets and carrots are done, remove from oven and allow to cool completely.
5. Add all ingredients for the Green Goddess dressing to the pitcher of a blender or food processor and blend until smooth. If the dressing is too thick slowly add more olive oil, 1 tablespoon at a time.
6. Once the beets are cooled, remove the skins using a small knife or peeler. Quarter beets and set aside.

(Extra prepared beets store great for salads. Keep them in your refrigerator for up to a week.)

7. On a platter arrange watercress, beets and carrots and drizzle with green goddess dressing. Top with micro greens and a little salt and freshly ground pepper and enjoy!

21. Tuna Salad and Chickpea Stuffed Avocado

Prep Time: 25 Minutes

Cook Time: 05 Minutes

Servings: 6

Ingredients

- 5 oz good quality tuna
- 4 tbsp plain greek yogurt
- 2 tsp olive oil
- 2 tsp za'atar
- 2 tsp lemon juice
- 1/3 cup chickpeas, drained, rinsed
- 1/2 tsp salt
- 1/2 tsp pepper
- 1/2 tsp garlic powder
- 1/2 tsp smoked paprika
- 2 large avocados, cut in half, pitted
- 1/2 cup loosely packed cilantro or micro greens
- 2 radishes, sliced
- 1/2 cup quick pickled onions

- 1/4 cup feta, crumbled
- 1/4 cup vegan chipotle sauce

Instructions

1. In a small bowl, mix the tuna with the yogurt, olive oil, za'atar, and lemon juice.
2. Place the chickpeas in a small bowl and season with the salt, pepper, garlic powder, and smoked paprika.
3. Fill the avocado halves with tuna salad, seasoned chickpeas, cilantro, radishes, quick pickled onions and feta. Top with vegan chipotle sauce and serve immediately.

Prep Time: 15 Minutes

Cook Time: 2hrs 25 Minutes

Servings: 8

Ingredients

- 1 lb dried red beans, rinsed
- 2 tbsp olive oil, divided
- 1 green bell pepper, chopped
- 1 medium yellow onion, chopped
- 1 cup celery, chopped
- 3 tbsp garlic, minced
- 1 large ham hock
- 1 tsp kosher salt
- 1/2 tsp freshly ground pepper
- 2 tsp fresh thyme (or 1/2 tsp dried)
- 3 bay leaves
- 2 tsp creole seasoning
- 2 tbsp flat leaf parsley, chopped (plus more for serving)
- 1 tbsp worcestershire sauce
- 1 lb smoked ham, diced

- 1/2 lb Andouille sausage, split in half lengthwise and cut into 1-inch pieces
- 1/2 Louisiana hot sausage, cut on the bias
- 1 jar pickled okra, for serving (optional)
- Louisiana hot sauce (like crystal), for serving (optional)
- 1 cooked white rice

Instructions

1. Place the beans in a large pot. Fill the pot of beans with water, double the beans volume. Bring to a boil. Boil the beans for 45 minutes making sure the beans are always covered in water. The beans should be tender with a little bite left in them.

2. While the beans are boiling, sauté celery, onion and bell pepper in 1 tablespoon olive oil in a large pan. When onions begin to soften add the garlic. Sauté until onions are translucent about 10 minutes. Set aside.

3. After the beans are done boiling, drain them and place the ham hock into the bottom of the pot. Add the onion-garlic mixture to the pot along with the beans. Add the salt, pepper, thyme, bay leaves,

Worcestershire sauce, parsley and Creole seasoning. Add just enough water to cover everything in the pot. Bring to a boil them simmer for 2-3 hours. During this time the beans will release starch which will turn the water and seasoning into a rich gravy. How "wet" the sauce is depends on your liking. If it gets too sticky, add water ¼ cup at a time.

4. While the red beans are melding with the deliciousness and making the sauce, add the last tablespoon of olive oil to the pan that was used for veggies. Sauté ham and sausage until slightly brown on all edges. During the last hour of simmering add it all to the pot of beans.

5. Serve over white rice along side pickled okra, Louisiana hot sauce and of course good corn bread.

6. Browning ham and sausage until crispy is completely optional if you're pressed for time. You'll still get great flavor, but we love the extra step as it crisps up the meat a little bit giving it a delicious texture!

7. If you have a leftover ham bone from the holidays, use it in place of the ham hock! Much better than split pea soup.

Prep Time: 10 Minutes

Cook Time: 25 Minutes

Servings: 4

Ingredients

- 4 cups cooked rice, preferably day old
- 3 large eggs, beaten
- 2 1/2 tsp toasted Sesame oil
- 1/3 cup Coconut aminos
- 1/4 tsp Salt, divided, plus more to taste 1/4 tsp
- 3-4 Tbsp Vegetable oil
- 2 medium carrots peeled and finely diced, about 1 cup
- 1/2 Medium onion, finely chopped, about 1 cup
- 3 Cloves garlic, minced
- 3/4 cup frozen peas
- 4 green onions, chopped
- 2-3 Tbsp soy sauce or Tamari

Instructions

1. If using freshly cooked rice (as opposed to day old) spread it out on a baking sheet or two large plates to cool.

2. In a small bowl beat the eggs together with ½ teaspoon sesame oil, 1/2 teaspoon coconut aminos and ¼ teaspoon salt.

3. Heat 1 tablespoon vegetable oil and 1 teaspoon sesame oil in a large saucepan or wok (if you have one) over medium heat. Add the carrots and cook for 3-4 minutes until slightly softening. Add the onions and cook for 4 minutes longer, until both onions and carrots are tender. Add the garlic to the pan and cook for 1 minute longer. Remove vegetables from the pan and set aside in a bowl.

4. Add 1 tablespoon of vegetable oil to the empty pan and quickly fry the eggs, moving them around until they're just set and there are no longer any wet parts. As soon as the eggs are cooked, take them out of the pan and add them to the bowl with the carrots and onions.

5. Add 1 tablespoon vegetable oil and 1 teaspoon sesame oil to the empty pan and fry the rice by spreading it in an even layer. Let the rice fry without disturbing it for

2-3 minutes at a time before tossing it and then frying it for another 2-3 minutes. Do this for a total of 3-4 times.

6. Add the carrot mixture to the pan along with the peas, eggs, green onions, remaining coconut aminos and soy sauce (or Tamari) to the pan and stir quickly over medium heat until it is all fully combined. Season to taste with salt.

7. We recommend cooking the rice at least 6 hours before making this dish or using day old previously cooked rice.

24. Chicken Street Tacos with Mango Slaw

Prep Time: 30 Minutes

Cook Time: 25 Minutes

Servings: 6

Ingredients

- 2 lbs boneless skinless chicken thighs
- 12-18 corn tortillas, street taco size, warmed
- 2 avocados, sliced
- tomatillo salsa, optional
- extra limes for serving, optional

Marinade:

- 1 orange, squeezed
- 1 lime, squeezed
- 6 cloves garlic, minced
- 2 tsp ancho chili powder
- 2 tsp onion powder
- 2 tsp smoked paprika
- 2 tsp salt
- 2 tsp pepper

Mango Slaw:

- 2 mangos, 1/2-inch diced
- 1/2 small red onion, minced or very thinly sliced
- 2 cups shredded red cabbage
- 1 cup cilantro leaves
- 2 limes, juiced
- salt to taste

Instructions

1. Mix all the marinade ingredients in a medium container fitted with a lid. Whisk or shake with lid on until fully incorporated. Add the chicken thighs and marinade at least 30 min or overnight if possible.

2. Heat oven to 425° F. Place the marinated chicken on a cooling or baking rack set on top of a rimmed baking sheet lined with foil. Cook the chicken until the internal temperature reaches 165° F, about 20 minutes.

3. In a large bowl mix the mangos, red onion, red cabbage, cilantro, the juice of two limes and salt to taste until combined.

4. Slice the chicken. Assemble the tacos by adding the chicken to warm tortillas, topped with mango slaw,

and sliced avocado. Serve with extra lime and tomatillo salsa if desired.

Prep Time: 20 Minutes

Cook Time: 40 Minutes

Servings: 4

Ingredients

- 2 lbs sirloin steaks, cut into 2-inch pieces
- 4 tbsp olive oil, divided
- 1 1/2 lb sweet potatoes, peeled and cut into 1-inch cubes
- 5 cloves garlic, minced
- 2 tsp salt
- cracked pepper
- Curry Aioli
- 3/4 cup good quality mayonnaise
- 1 clove garlic minced
- 1 tsp curry powder

Instructions

1. In a small bowl mix together mayonnaise, garlic and curry powder until smooth and set aside.

2. Heat 2 tablespoons olive oil in a large cast iron skillet over medium-high heat. Add the sweet potatoes to the pan in single layer. Let sit untouched for 3-5 minutes until golden brown. Toss in the pan for an additional 10-12 minutes until fork tender. Remove from pan and set aside.

3. Season steak pieces generously with salt and pepper.

4. Heat 2 tbsp of olive oil over high heat. Add in steak bites in a single layer, making sure they aren't touching each other. Cook on high untouched until steak bites are well browned, turn sides and repeat. Continue cooking until all sides are brown. If working in batches, remove the first batch from the pan and cook the remaining steak.

5. Once all the steak is cooked add both sweet potatoes and all steak back into the pan along with the garlic and cook for 1-2 minutes until garlic is fragrant.

6. Serve hot with curry aioli.

Prep Time: 15 Minutes

Cook Time: 35 Minutes

Servings: 6

Ingredients

- 1 Tbsp olive oil
- 1 medium yellow onion, diced
- 3 cloves garlic, minced
- 1 Tbsp fresh ginger, minced
- 3 Tbsp yellow curry powder
- 2 tsp cinnamon
- 2 tsp cumin
- 2 tsp sea salt
- 1 (14oz) can diced tomatoes
- 3 (14oz) cans coconut milk, unsweetened
- 1 large head of cauliflower, cut into bite-sized florets
- cilantro (otpional)
- naan (optional)
- rice (optional)

Instructions

1. In a 5-quart (or medium-sized stock pot) heat olive oil over medium heat. Add onions and sauté until translucent, about 5 minutes. Add the garlic and ginger and continue sautéing until fragrant, about 1 minute.

2. Stir in the curry powder, cinnamon, cumin, salt and tomatoes.

3. Stir in coconut milk and bring the pot to a boil. Simmer for 5 minutes, stirring often.

4. Use an immersion blender to blend the curry mixture until smooth. Alternatively, remove from heat, transfer the curry to a blender, blending until smooth.

5. Return the pot to a boil and add the cauliflower florets. Simmer until the cauliflower is fork-tender, about 15 minutes.

6. Serve over rice with with fresh cilantro and warm naan.

Prep Time: 20 Minutes

Cook Time: 15 Minutes

Servings: 4

Ingredients

- 1 lb ground chorizo
- 1 (15 oz) can refried beans
- 8 tostada shells, store-bought or homemade
- 1/2 cup crumbled cotija cheese
- 2 cups shredded iceberg lettuce
- 1/2 cup pico de gallo
- 1 cup guacamole
- 1 lime, cut into 8 wedges

White Sauce:

- 1/2 cup sour cream
- 2 tsp lime juice
- 1/2 tsp dried oregano
- 1/4 tsp salt
- 1/2 tsp ground cumin
- 1/2 tsp garlic powder

- Mexican hot sauce, to taste (such as Tapatio)
- 1 Tbsp milk, optional

Instructions

1. In a large skillet set over medium heat, cook the chorizo, crumbling it with a wooden spoon, about 5-6 minutes.
2. While the chorizo is cooking, make the white sauce. In a small bowl or small food processor combine all ingredients and blend until smooth. Add milk, a little at a time, until desired consistency is achieved.
3. When the chorizo is fully cooked, add the refried beans to the skillet, mixing with the chorizo until fully combined and warmed through.
4. Spread the warm meat and bean mixture onto the tostada shells. Sprinkle with cotija cheese, iceberg lettuce, pico de gallo, guacamole and more cotija.
5. Drizzle the finished tostada with desired amount white sauce, a squeeze of lime and hot sauce.

Prep Time: 10 Minutes

Cook Time: 20 Minutes

Servings: 6

Ingredients

- 1 1/2 cups plain breadcrumbs
- 2 tsp sea salt
- 1 1/2 tsp sugar
- 3/4 tsp paprika (not smoked)
- 3/4 tsp onion powder
- 3/4 tsp garlic powder
- 1/2 tsp black pepper
- pinch of cayenne, optional
- 1 tsp dried basil, oregano or parsley (any combination of these will work)
- 1/4 cup vegetable oil
- 3 lbs boneless, skinless chicken breast (about 6), 3 lbs of chicken breast tenders or 6 (1/2 inch thick) bone-in or boneless pork chops.

Instructions

1. Heat the oven to 400°F.

2. Combine the breadcrumbs, salt, sugar, paprika, onion powder, garlic powder, black pepper, cayenne and your choice of dried herbs in a large zip-top bag. Seal the bag and toss the spice mixture until combined.

3. Open the bag, drizzle in the oil. Seal the bag and mix again until the oil is fully incorporated.

4. Fill a medium-sized bowl or pie pan with a little water. Working with one chicken breast or pork chop at a time, moisten the meat with the water, allowing any excess to drip off back into the pan. This will help the spiced breadcrumb mixture adhere to the meat.

5. One at a time, add the pieces of chicken or pork to the bag of seasoned breadcrumbs. Add one piece, seal the bag and shake until the meat is completely covered in breadcrumbs. Open the bag and move the crumb-coated meat to an ungreased or foil-covered rimmed baking sheet. Repeat with remaining pieces or meat.

6. Cook until the internal temperature of the meat is where it's supposed to be when checked with an instant-read thermometer—165° F for chicken or 145°F for pork chops. It will take about 15-20 minutes,

depending on the thickness of your meat. Do not cover or turn the meat while baking.

Prep Time: 15 Minutes

Cook Time: 45 Minutes

Servings: 8

Ingredients

- 1/2 cup butter (1 stick)
- 2 cups carrots, 1/4 inch sliced
- 1 cup celery, 1/4 inch sliced
- 1 cup onion, chopped
- 1/2 cup flour
- 1 tsp salt
- 1/2 tsp black pepper
- 1/2 tsp celery seed
- 1 tsp garlic powder
- 1 tsp fresh thyme, minced (optional)
- 1 cup whole milk
- 2 cups chicken stock
- 2 cups peas, frozen
- 4 cups cooked chicken (3 chicken breasts, pre cooked or rotisserie)
- 1 package frozen puff pastry, slightly thawed

- 1 egg (for pastry wash)

Instructions

1. Heat oven to 425°F.

2. Melt the butter in a 12" inch cast iron (or other oven proof) skillet over medium heat. Add the onion, celery, carrots to the butter and sauté for 5 minutes, until the onions are tender and translucent.

3. Add the flour, salt, pepper, celery seed, garlic powder and thyme to the butter and vegetables creating a thick paste. Sauté for 2 minutes.

4. Slowly add the milk. Once the milk is fully incorporated, slowly add the chicken stock. Simmer, whisking continuously until mixture has slightly thickened.

5. Add the peas and chicken to the sauce.

6. Roll out one pastry sheet into a 16-inch square on a lightly floured surface. Cut into 26 (3-inch) squares. Place the squares, slightly overlapping on top of the chicken mixture.

7. In a small bowl, whisk the egg with 1 tbsp water. Brush the egg wash over the puff pastry. Place in the oven for 25 minutes until pastry is golden brown and

filling is bubbling. If it is browning too quickly, cover with foil after it gets as dark as you'd like.

Prep Time: 15 Minutes

Cook Time: 25 Minutes

Servings: 4

Ingredients

- 1.5 lb Salmon fillet, cut into 4 pieces
- 4 large carrots, peeled and cut into into 3" matchsticks
- 3 cups broccoli florets
- 1 tbsp brown sugar
- 1 tsp sesame oil
- ½ cup low sodium soy sauce or tamari
- ¼ cup cilantro, minced
- 1 tsp ginger, minced
- 2 tsp garlic, minced
- 1 tbsp sesame seeds
- 4 green onions, minced, optional

Instructions

1. Preheat oven to 400°F.

2. In a small bowl, combine brown sugar, sesame oil, soy sauce or tamari, cilantro, ginger, garlic and sesame seeds.

3. On a large baking sheet, arrange salmon fillets, broccoli and carrots. Drizzle half of the sauce over the entire sheet pan, using your hands to toss if needed.

4. Bake on center rack for 18 minutes.

5. Drizzle with remaining sauce, sprinkle with green onions and serve warm along with rice or just as is.